The ¾ Rule

How To Eat As

A Young Athlete

CHRIS WEILER

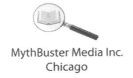

MythBuster Media Inc.
Chicago

Books may be purchased in quantity and/or special sales
by contacting the publisher.

MythBuster Media Inc.
Chicago
sales@MythBusterMedia.com
www.MythBusterMedia.com

Library of Congress Control Number: 2013909609

ISBN 0989179605
ISBN 978-0-9891796-0-7
Cover Design: Gion-Per Marxer - Gion-Per@BeeCoding.com

Contents

Acknowledgements

To my mother, for introducing me at a young age to smarter nutrition and to question everything.

To my wife Ronda, for being my constant cheerleader, even when you think I'm crazy.

To my daughter Isabelle, for your valuable input and perspective as a young athlete - You Rock!

To Carol, always thoughtful and supportive.

To Marcie, for your guidance on language and colors.

To Russ, for your voice of reason and feedback.

Thank You!

Preface

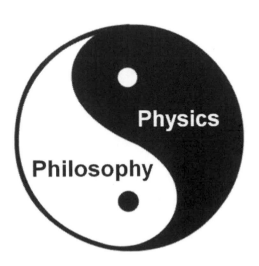

My background is in philosophy and physics. Simply put, philosophy is the science of how to think about things and physics is the science of how things work. Continuing my education through the National Academy of Sports Medicine provided a lens for me to focus and apply my background in how to develop the body. My objective is to generally teach *how to think* about how nutrition works and to specifically teach *how to eat* as a developing athlete.

How did my interest in this area begin? Well, one summer day before I entered eighth grade, I read multiple articles on exercise and nutrition. Two things happened as a result.

First, I stood up from the table and declared to my family that I would stop using salt. And second, I rode my bike 6 ½ miles the next day to join the nearest health club and never looked back.

That summer I completely changed my diet, including forming a lifelong relationship with protein and becoming a regular at the local health food store. Think 800 square foot mom and pop store, as Whole Foods did not yet exist. Being a student of nutrition has enabled me to witness, research, and experiment with virtually every nutrition and eating methodology devised over the past 30 years.

The ¾ Rule exists inside a larger Performance Model I created for athletic development. It begins with assessments to discover what is weak or imbalanced (restricted) in each athlete. This process is followed by four phases of development where those restrictions are addressed. The focus of this book is part of phase one: **Nutrition for Athletes.** I will explain exactly how young athletes should eat to support their bodies for practice, games and development.

I'm passionate about investigating how our bodies work and creating Performance Models that make it easy for others to understand the insights I've gained. In helping develop young athletes for most major sports, I am often asked, "What should my child eat for peak performance?" When I applied my Performance Model to come up with an answer, I realized the wrong question was being asked. The relevant question is "*How* should my child eat?"

The ¾ **Rule** was born out of my passion to provide a rock-solid nutrition model guided by a few simple rules. I want to reduce the stress and wasted time associated with trying to keep up with the latest nutrition flavor of the moment. Unlike most "experts," I don't provide tips, tricks or "things to try." Just like The Scientific Model, **The ¾ Rule** is a model that provides a methodology within a flexible framework that can accommodate everyone's needs.

One model, one rule – everyone's nutrition needs met.

The secret, whether we are talking math, linguistics, geology, music, or physical development, is education. On the cellular level, our bodies are indifferent to whether we are attempting to develop our foreign language skills or our basketball skills. In both cases, the body uses the same pathways of communication, the nervous system and one model: stimulation, response, adaptation.

The engine that drives my Performance Model is an education model that teaches you *how* to think about the correct development of the body. When you understand *how* to think about development, you can use that thought process to correctly apply the tools and rules in the model. Knowing *how* to do something powers *what* you are doing and is the magic in an education-driven model – empowerment!

These are the circumstances that shaped my mission
"Powerful Athletes and Healthy Bodies for Life!"

Disclaimer - You know, the legal stuff

This book is not intended to take the place of your personal physician's/pediatrician's advice. It is not intended to diagnose, treat, cure or prevent any disease or dysfunction. Discuss this information with your own physician or healthcare provider to determine what is right for you.

Remember, every individual has their own unique genetic, biological, physiological, neurological and metabolic markers, variances, tolerances, considerations and predispositions. Therefore, you should FIRST always consult with your medical doctor to make sure anything written or suggested in this book, a particular food and/or supplement is not contraindicated for you specifically.

Introduction

It's Monday morning and your ten-year-old son, Caden, who plays football, soccer and basketball, wakes up late for school. He "doesn't have time for breakfast." His first meal of the day is lunch – typically a low nutrient-value experience because it is not balanced. Right after school he has sports practice.

Meanwhile, that same morning, his twelve-year-old competitive gymnast sister Isabelle has time to eat but emphatically says, "I can't eat in the morning; it makes me sick." Although Isabelle brings her lunch to school, she typically throws it out except for the treat/desert portion. *Many parents are unaware of this very common practice.* The result is that both scenarios add up to a very poor recipe for developing minds and bodies.

Traffic is slow and your son's coach needs to speak with you for a few minutes. Now you are running late which means there is no time to get a proper meal before Isabelle's 3-4 hour gymnastics practice. *Thankfully* there is a fast food establishment nearby where you can buy doughnuts and beverages to dunk them in, along with an assortment of high fat, high carbohydrate, low protein sandwiches. Sure, it's better than nothing in a pinch, but not as a rule for proper development.

Finally, it's time for dinner. This is often the first opportunity in nearly twenty-four hours for a complete, nutrient-dense meal. However, Isabelle says, "I'm not hungry. I'm tired, need to shower and have like, 2 hours of homework."

For many young athletes and parents I speak with, this dynamic often becomes the rule rather than the exception.

As responsible parents we don't compromise our expectations on academic development; they must go to school, do their homework, and earn certain grades. Although some kids don't enjoy school, and if given the choice many kids would choose not to go to school, they know this is not an option. Our kids must go to school, do their homework, brush their teeth and wear appropriate clothing for the weather. So why do we pay more attention to what happens outside of their bodies rather than what they put inside their bodies? When it comes to our kids' physical or athletic development, we negotiate, compromise, and take the path of least resistance on a regular basis.

Imagine for a moment that from a very young age, both Isabelle and Caden were simply raised with the understanding that academic and physical development are both equal, non-negotiable ingredients that support their complete development. Idealistic fantasy? Maybe not. Since we learn what we live, all this requires is for the entire family to make nutrition a priority and to be on the same page. This does not mean that every family member must eat exactly the same foods, but rather have all family members apply one nutritional model to their individual lives. We already accept and apply this dynamic to education in that some family members may be in AP courses, while others may need an IEP. Everyone is having their individual academic needs met under the umbrella of one objective – education.

Probably the most significant difference between the academic and physical realms is that we send our kids to school where there are "experts" to address their academic development while their physical development is left to the non-expert – *you*.

Sports do not adequately address physical development. Coaches teach fundamentals, skills, game play, strategy and teamwork. However, this has little to do with building a strong physical foundation to support the development of those sport-specific skills. It also doesn't address the prevention of imbalances and acute/chronic injuries in order to promote healthy bodies for life. This is important, as the leading cause of youth sports injuries by far (74%) is musculoskeletal imbalance. This is more significant than the damage caused by impact injuries, including concussions, breaks, and fractures.

And as little as coaches know about athletic development, they often know considerably less about the role of nutrition. Typically, this holds true for you as well. Since you bear the responsibility for your child's nutrition, you need a simple, powerful tool that you can immediately integrate into your lifestyle in any environment. Although this book is focused on nutrition for young athletes, what I will show you next is a model for nutrition that can easily apply to all family members (athletes or couch potatoes) and shows you exactly *how* to eat as an athlete and for life.

The ¾ Rule.

Let's dig in!

Chapter 1

Why Athletes Need Food

I believe in applying the efficiency principle in all areas of life and this book is no exception. For this reason I will get right to the point of why you are reading a book about nutrition for athletes. You believe nutrition is important and want to make sure you, your child or if you're a coach/trainer your athletes are eating properly. So you know what you want but don't know

HOW IT WORKS.

Life's short and I respect your time. So unlike most nutrition books I'm going to give you what you came for up front - right now. After you learn "Why Athletes Need Food" and discover how to apply **The 3/4 Rule** you will have 2 options.

1. Close the book, apply **The 3/4 Rule** and never look back.
2. Continue reading to understand exactly why Nutrition for Athletes works, what it's based on and the thinking that supports the model.

Why Athletes Need Food

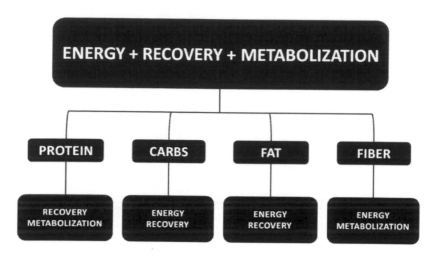

As this chart illustrates, athletes need food for *energy*, *recovery* and *metabolization*. Our bodies convert our food into energy through metabolization, which is just a fancy word for how our body breaks down food and gives it to the parts of the body that need it.

Referring to the chart you will notice that we are only concerned with 4 general nutrients from our food: protein, carbohydrates, fat and fiber – period. What about phytonutrients, macro/micro nutrients, anti-oxidants, fatty acids, etc? When you follow a powerful model like **The 3/4 Rule**, you don't have to sweat the details. Simply follow **The ¾ Rule** and all your nutrition needs will be met.

Chapter 2

The ¾ Rule

The **3/4 Rule** is the engine that drives Nutrition for Athletes and its crazy simple. The graphic represents your meal plate where 3/4 of your plate should be filled with *protein* from meat, fish or eggs and *carbohydrates* from a combination of whole grains, vegetables, beans and/or fruit.

You don't count calories or worry about fat. You also do not have to eat from all four carbohydrate groups every meal, but at some point during the day you should have servings from each group.

What about serving sizes or portions? It doesn't matter how much or little you consume at any one meal because the ratios are what is important as our bodies require balance. Your plate should be visually in balance. So a 16oz steak with a mouthful of rice and a bite of lettuce is NOT in balance. However, for some people at some meals, all you need is a couple bites of protein and carbohydrates to satisfy the Rule.

I just said don't worry about serving sizes, but some of you are thinking right now, *"how much protein should I eat per day?"* The simplest guideline to follow is about half your body weight in grams per day. If you weigh 150lbs then eat around 75grams of protein per day. For reference, a 3 - 4 oz piece of meat/fish has about 25 grams of protein. Do some people need more/less - yes. The longer and more intensely you train your body, the more protein most people need for proper energy, recovery and metabolization.

Yes, at minimum you need to eat breakfast, lunch and dinner. Feel free to eat more frequently, but you MUST eat these three meals as regularly as possible.

Now at this point some of you are wrestling with objections I simply refer to as your *circumstances*.

- OMG! I can't eat in the morning, especially protein.
- I hate fish, eggs, meat, beans, fruit, etc.
- I'm vegan, raw, etc.
- We don't do leftovers.
- What about soy, nut butters, milk, etc.
- I'm too tired to eat when I get home from practice.
- I don't have time, too much homework, etc.

While I completely validate your personal *circumstances* your body is indifferent to them. On the cellular level, your body's metabolic processes are tasked with precise instructions; extract specific nutrients from food and transport them to the parts of the body that need it – period.

To be clear, clinging tightly to your *circumstances* is okay, but your *circumstances* do not invalidate **The 3/4 Rule.** You need to decide if supporting your *circumstances* is worth interfering with your athletic development.

You're body is either getting the nutrients it needs for proper energy, recovery and metabolization or it is not. If your body is not getting the nutrients it needs there are automatic consequences that will hurt you as an athlete. Cause and effect baby – nobody is immune.

CHEW ON THIS!

Can you apply this to every meal, of course not, but you can always keep it in mind and apply it to as many meals as possible.

Integration in the home

Although integrating a new eating dynamic in the home can be a challenge, if done right it can further strengthen your family's bonds. Kids often don't like to be singled out even for things they like.

In 2004, the mother of a child I began training asked me to also help with her child's nutrition. When I asked about their current eating dynamic, the rest of the family ate a lot of packaged *grab food* and often had pizza and hot dogs for dinner. Her child's nutrition plan would most likely have failed if the rest of the family did not accept that they needed to approach this as a family, a team. I said, 'have a family discussion where you explain that we, as a team, are all going to be adopting a new way of eating to help us feel, look and play great.'

By using this approach, they created an empowering support system for each other while forging another positive relational anchor point within their family.

The point: don't read this book and say to your child, "here's what YOU need to do." Be a team!

This is a great topic to discuss in more detail online.
Go to www.ChrisWeiler.com/Nutrition
or Scan the QR code below with your mobile device.

Keep it simple

I want to make sure you are absolutely clear on how simple it is to apply **The 3/4 Rule**. Simply split 3/4 of your plate in half and fill it with protein and carbohydrates from the listed sources. Your protein and carbohydrate servings should take up about the same amount of space as each other on 3/4 of your plate - period.

Rest assured, **The 3/4 Rule** is not restrictive. It simply takes the same food we all have access to and plugs it into a structure that maximally supports physical development. You will still find a huge variety of food to choose from that you enjoy, have access to and can afford.

In following this model you will get everything you need to support *Nutrition for Survival* and *Nutrition for Athletes*. We'll discuss the distinction in a later chapter, but for now you are almost done learning **The 3/4 Rule!**

The ¾ Rule

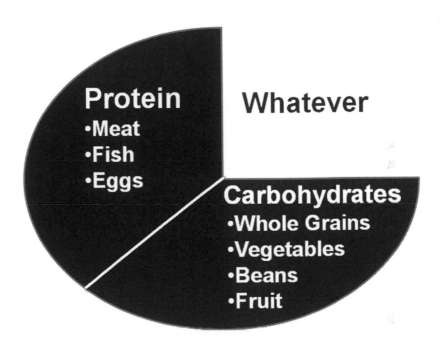

Now some of you observant folks may have noticed that there was a quarter missing in **The 3/4 Rule**. The last 1/4 is called "Whatever". That means you have the option of filling in the last 1/4 of your plate with pizza, a cookie, a slice of pie, a candy bar – Whatever! The only rule is that it must be in relative proportion with the other 3/4 of your plate. This means if you have a 3oz piece of fish, 2 tablespoons of brown rice and a bite or two of broccoli, you cannot fill the last 1/4 of your plate with 6 brownies - It's not in proportion. GOT IT?!

Your plate should be in "visual proportion." If you look at your plate with a reasonable mind you know what looks visually in balance or in proportion and what does not. Relax, this is not an exact measurement; it's more of a visual estimation.

CHEW ON THIS!

It's not a requirement that you fill the last 1/4 of your plate with some nutritionally bankrupt, artificially flavored, sugar packed food; you could fill it with a piece of fruit, vegetable... or nothing.

While preparing for my first presentation on The 3/4 Rule, it was my 11 year old competitive gymnast daughter who said to me, "you need to make "Whatever" more specific, because you know what some kids are going to do...?" 'What' I asked.' "If you don't qualify "Whatever" some kids are going to stack 8 pieces of pizza or doughnuts on top of one another in that 1/4 space on their plate – I know I would." Although both my daughter and wife agree that my stop age is around 14, it never occurred to me that the loophole in **The 3/4 Rule** was to stack my food vertically in the 1/4 space. Brilliant - but oh so wrong.

So, I have closed the loophole with "In Relative Proportion" or "Visual Proportion."

*Nuts and seeds (typically viewed as fruit) should be included on the carbohydrate side as their protein is incomplete. Since many schools and teams ban nuts due to allergies, I have not include them, but you may if you choose.

CHEW ON THIS!

The 3/4 Rule *is a tool and as such the skill in which you apply this tool is dependent on your intentions. Your mind guides how you use the tool, which in turn determines the quality of what you are trying to build. If you have a self-defeating perspective then you will be looking for opportunities and excuses to not use the tool correctly and therefore not achieve your objectives.*

A NOTE ABOUT MILK

Milk should NOT be counted as a protein for athletes, which begs the question, what side of the plate does it go on? Let's treat all milk except flavored milk as independent of **The 3/4 Rule.** Drink as little or as much milk as you like for taste and calcium, without it being considered at all in regards to **The 3/4 Rule.** Flavored milk is the exception due to its high sugar content and therefore belongs in the ¼ portion of your plate at any given meal.

I know... Don't count milk as protein is *fightin'* words. I fully explain myself in Chapter 6 – All Protein is Not Created Equal.

A NOTE ABOUT CHOCOLATE MILK

Recovery Drinks are to replenish glycogen in muscles due to intense, prolonged training such as training for a triathlon.

If you run for 90+ minutes in the morning followed by biking and swimming for 90+ minutes later that same day, then chocolate milk has been found to do a better job as a recovery tool than sugary sports drinks. However, if you train below this threshold of time and intensity, which includes most athletes, then chocolate milk is the wrong tool for the job.

Have Questions? Comments? Continue the discussion online. www.ChrisWeiler.com/Nutrition

Or scan QR code with QR Reader application on your mobile device.

That's it my friends - you're done!

That's the Nutrition for Athletes Model! I told you it was easy. Simply apply **The 3/4 Rule** as often as possible and you will be giving your body the exact ingredients it needs to support your athletic development recipe.

If all you came here for was the Nutrition for Athletes Model and how to apply **The 3/4 Rule**, you're done – enjoy. If you are interested in learning why and the thinking that supports the model, please continue reading.

Chapter 3

"Give a fish – Feed for a day.

Teach to fish – Feed for Life!"

This well known concept illustrates the difference between the *what* and the *how*. In the quoted concept of this chapter title, the objective is to help someone acquire food to eat – the *what*. But if I give you a fish, that only feeds you for today, what about when you get hungry tomorrow? You see by just giving you the *what*, I haven't actually taught you *how* to get your objective met. What happens if I move, die or simply don't feel like giving you a fish today; how will you meet your eating objectives then? This is why it is vital we understand that *how* we do something is usually much more powerful and important in making lasting changes in our lives than *what* we do.

There are often many paths we can take to meet an objective, but our success usually lies in how we apply ourselves while navigating those paths rather than what path we choose.

The "*thing*" Has No Power!

You Do!

It is for this reason that both my personal and business philosophy are driven by The "*thing*" Has No Power!

In our tech driven, push button society we love to give our power for accomplishing tasks to "*things*" - our pads, pods and phones; push that big red "Easy Button" and all your office supply needs will be met.

Most of us ask the same question regarding nutrition – "What should I eat?" This is because we are conditioned to give power to the "*thing*" the food. Instead the question ought to be "How should I eat?"

You see the *how* helps determine *what* you should eat.

The fantasy marketed, advertised and sold to our conditioned minds is that there are magic exercises, equipment and food that will automatically grant us our goals and objectives if they are used and/or consumed, but this simply is not true.

Although beyond the scope of this book, there is not one diet or eating plan for weight loss that has EVER existed that does not work by the exact same principle – calories in, calories out. That's right, I don't care what label you slap on that diet; liquid, grapefruit, raw, points, prepared meals, blood type, high protein/fat, low carbs, caveman, etc. all have the same engine under the hood. You see when you scrape off the slick shiny layers of marketing goo, the exposed core at its chewy center is calories in, calories out – period. It's just a matter of *how* you apply yourself and the tools you are using that determine your success.

A Nutrition Policy That Ensures Success

This is why it is important I teach you *How to Eat* as an athlete and not *What to Eat*. I can't possibly know each of your likes, dislikes, allergies, budgets, or religious circumstances that can affect food choice. What about when you eat at grandmas next week, go to a new restaurant or out of town? You see when you use a proper policy, practice or model of *how* to do something you cover everyone for any future circumstances that you could not possibly imagine at the present – That's the power of a strong model.

The Scientific Model (Method) is an example of a model many people have a frame of reference for. From hypothesis and experimentation to results and conclusion, everyone looking to conduct a valid experiment follows the Scientific Model. Along with the subject matter of your experiment, your background, experiences, credentials, title, published works, ethnicity, religion and/or ego are completely irrelevant.

The Scientific Model provides a framework that guides one in "How" to conduct a valid experiment. This framework is infinitely flexible in that it can accommodate any experiment and if the rules of the model are followed and applied correctly, you will produce valid results.

In this same spirit I created **The 3/4 Rule** as a model to guide the proper Nutrition for Young Athletes. Simply follow the rules in the model and all your nutrition needs as an athlete will be met. Actually, all your nutrition needs will be met whether you are an athlete or not. However, for the purposes of this book I am specifically applying this model to young athletes.

Chapter 4

"Nutrition for Survival"

What Your Body Cares About

- Brain
- Heart
- Intestines
- Kidneys
- Liver
- Lungs
- Stomach

Nutrition for Survival is what your body cares about which is to keep you alive.

On the cellular level your body is not concerned with your personal objectives. It does not care that you want to be stronger, faster, win your league championship, make varsity, get an athletic scholarship, etc. – it merely responds to stimulus. As such it is tasked with making sure your heart is beating, lungs are respiring, kidneys filtering and flushing, you get the idea.

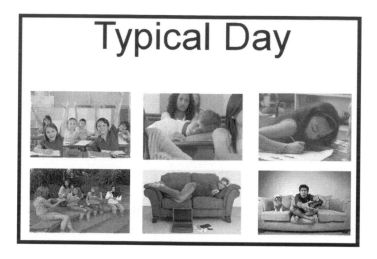

The image above illustrates a typical day in the life of our youth. With the exception of extracurricular activities, these represent what the majority of kids experience throughout any given week. Go to school, maybe take a nap, do some homework, hang out with friends, zone out to the TV or get your game on.

At some point during these activities you're going to get...

HUNGRY!

Hunger is one of the body's survival alarms, trying to communicate to you that it's running low on its fuel, nutrients from food. Your body sounds the hunger alarm so it can fulfill its primary objective – keeping you alive.

Many of us have been told that you should only eat when you are hungry as a sensible way to manage caloric intake. After all, the body is smart, it knows when it needs food and tells you– makes sense in your head, right?

The answer is no. What we find is that our hunger alarm is designed to help us survive; which means it is part of Nutrition for Survival and not necessarily Nutrition for Athletes. Nutrition for Survival, merely keeping you alive, has little to do in support of your sports performance objectives.

CHEW ON THIS!

Sometimes athletes need to eat when they are NOT hungry. Your body needs repair materials from food whether you feel like eating or not. Relax, follow **The 3/4 Rule** *and just have few bites of protein and carbohydrates and you're good to go.*

"Nutrition for Athletes"

What YOU Need to Care About

Energy and Recovery beyond "Nutrition for Survival"

Nutrition for Athletes is what you need to care about; energy and recovery beyond Nutrition for Survival. This supports activities such as those you see illustrated above, which I think you will agree are very different than the activities you see pictured below.

Typical Day

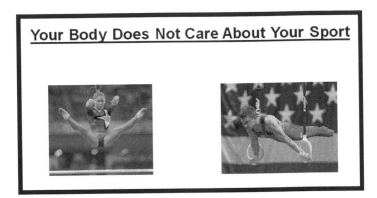

The images above are of two Olympic gymnasts Shawn Johnson and Jonathan Horton. Do you think that perhaps the energy requirements of these athletes and their activities are different than the requirements of this poor little guy illustrated below?

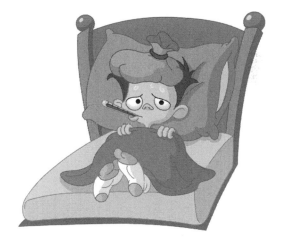

So it's important to look at the quality of survival when deciding how to feed your body. In the examples below, both the gymnasts and the boy in bed are surviving, but the nutritional requirements needed to support their survival are quite different.

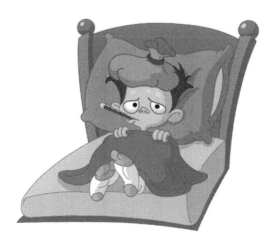

Your Body Does Not Care About Your Sport

Maybe we should consider this in terms of surviving versus thriving. The body needs very little nutrition to merely survive. History is replete with cultures that have survived on very little or one main food source that did not provide complete nutrients. These people may be weak, malnourished and in poor health, but they survive.

To thrive however, athletes, especially young developing ones need complete balanced nutrition in the form of proper Proteins, Whole Grains, Vegetables, Beans and Fruit.

Now I know some of you caught that I qualified the protein above as "proper" so let's address that now.

Chapter 5

All protein is not created equal

All protein is not created equal, so the protein sources you choose make a difference in the quality of your development. We are what we eat is true in the sense that about every 6 months we replace a large percentage of the cells in our body – blood, skin, hair, etc. As such, the nutrients we put in our body literally help shape our future selves.

For a protein to be complete it must contain all *9 essential amino acids in correct proportion to one another*. Therefore, meat, fish, eggs, dairy, quinoa, soy and soybean based products such as tofu, are all complete proteins and not much else.

For you vegans out there, although some plant based proteins have all 9 amino acids, they are not all in sufficient quantities to satisfy the requirement of "correct proportion" to be considered a "complete" protein.

However, even "complete" proteins are not all created equal. Dairy, soy, soybean, tofu, and quinoa are fine for Nutrition for Survival, but not preferred protein sources for athletes. Yes they will do in a pinch invoking the "it's better than nothing" principle.

Although some athletes do just fine on a vegan diet, most do not. Everyone has their own unique biochemical soup and sometimes, for whatever reason, their biochemistry is such that it can satisfy that individual's protein needs with non meat protein sources. Remember, exceptions do not invalidate the rule or represent the average or majority; that is why they are called exceptions.

IT'S NOT ENOUGH

By law, most milk products sold in the U.S. as food must be pasteurized to kill harmful organisms. Raw milk may not be sold or transported across state lines. The problem is that this heat pasteurization process also destroys a number of enzymes which fracture the essential amino acid profile lowering its actual available protein. How low, we don't know. To be fair, there is evidence that the protein loss is only about 1-2 grams. Not a lot in itself, but a large percentage of what it can maximally offer per serving.

Add to this each individual's greater or lesser capacity to absorb the net available protein and then metabolize and distribute it to the needy parts of the body and your theoretical potential 8g of protein per 8oz of dairy is reduced to something less.

Since there are proponents on both sides of the pasture regarding viable protein after pasteurization let's discuss this next.

The three metrics used to measure protein in food and their effects on humans are Biological Value (BV), Protein Efficiency Rating (PER) and Protein Digestibility Corrected Amino Acid Score (PDCAAS). Each have their pros and cons and therefore the only thing science can agree on is that each is flawed and each does not provide a complete picture.

This is another opportunity to help teach you how to think about Nutrition for Athletes. How do we make correct decisions today when science does not have the answers? We move from what we know as fact and build on it using reason to form correct conclusions.

Fact: Heat destroys enzymes and protein.

Fact: Pasteurization is the process of heating dairy to kill harmful organisms.

Fact: Most milk in U.S. is pasteurized as it's illegal to sell or transport raw milk across state lines.

Therefore: The protein in the majority of dairy products sold in the U.S. has been compromised to some degree due to the effects of pasteurization.

Technically, pasteurization "denatures" proteins. In this context, denatured is just a fancy word for altering the chemical structure of proteins which renders some of them biologically inactive.

Wait a minute! Don't we "pasteurize" meat, eggs and fish when we cook them? You bet! So this is not a question of pasteurization being evil; remember The *"thing"* Has No Power! This is an issue of what is being pasteurized.

Low Start Values

Simply put, dairy has a low protein start value.

Dairy products have a protein start value of 8g per serving, while a serving of meat and fish have a start value of around 25g. Both will serve Nutrition for Survival where lower protein intake is not an issue, but is a great detriment to developing athletes and therefore is not sufficient to support Nutrition for Athletes.

The harder and more frequently athletes train and practice, especially strength train, the more damage is done to their tissues. For the young athlete this is compounded by the demands of developmental growth cycles, raging hormones, school/homework and as a result typically poor sleep/recovery cycles.

This tissue damage and lifestyle dynamic require raw repair materials in the form of protein, carbohydrates and fats – especially protein. Simply put, the more damage and stress to your system, the more nutrient repair materials needed. This is why protein start value is so important, especially for young developing athletes.

Hold your horses there bub! Don't eggs also have a low protein start value? It's true. Depending on the size of the egg, its start value is between 5-8g per egg, very similar to dairy.

The difference is in *How* we actually consume eggs, dairy and meat versus the stated serving size. A serving of dairy is 8oz – a glass of milk. A serving of eggs is 1 egg and a serving of meat or fish is around 3.5oz.

A glass of milk, the stated serving size is reasonable. However, although there are 15 year old boys who walk in the house and down a half gallon of milk with dinner, it's by no means the majority and certainly even fewer girls. So you can't count on your child consuming a large enough volume of milk to compensate for its low protein start value.

Conversely, very few people consume just one egg at a sitting. Between 2-4 eggs covers what most people actually consume, which means we need to multiply the serving size by how many eggs actually consumed. When we do this we have an adjusted protein start value between 13–32g.* This assumes large and extra large eggs as a reference point since these are the most common size eggs purchased. *And on a practical note, hard boiled eggs are much easier to transport for practices and games than milk.*

When considering meat and fish, the start value issue is compounded further as many people of all ages consume at least 3.5oz of meat or fish and often more at a given meal.

*For reference, a large egg has 6-7g of protein and an extra large egg has 7-8g of protein.

CHEW ON THIS!

Drink all the milk you want; bathe in it if you like. I just don't recommend it as one of your main protein sources to support Nutrition for Athletes.

I'll say it again...

1) Low protein start value.

2) Most people do not consume enough to compensate for the low protein start value.

I hope you are beginning to see the difference between the *what* and the *how* and why The *"thing"* Has No Power! I could tote the party line, echo everyone else and say "drink milk, it's a complete and good protein source." But milk technically being a protein source is not relevant or very useful if you cannot consume enough to meet your protein requirements.

I am trying to share with you the empowerment that goes along with *How* to think about these things. My intention is to help relieve some of the stress associated with our technology heavy, information overload lifestyles. Coaches and parents of young athletes spend way too much time navigating the endless waves of information and latest training and nutrition flavors of the moment in trying to support the care and feeding of their athletic youth.

Keep it simple. Follow The 3/4 Rule.

Chapter 6

How to Decode Nutrition Labels

I'll say it again; The *"thing"* Has No Power! We can't give our power to what the manufacturers tell us through their nutrition labels or ingredients list. This is giving power to the information and information can be twisted, spun and served up to you any way the manufacturer sees fit.

Serving size is completely made up by the manufacturer and is in large part tied to its total calories, fat and/or carbohydrate content. If a manufacturer thinks its consumers may be sensitive to a high calorie number and/or higher fat/carbohydrates then they will make the serving size smaller so it reflects fewer calories, grams of fat and carbohydrates.

Here is how the game is played. A consumer advocacy group such as Center for Science in the Public Interest lobbies hard to force congress to pass legislation such as the mandatory nutrition disclosure labels on most food items.

(Yes, in large part we have CSPI to thank for our nutrition labels. By the way, this group produces an amazing nutrition publication called Nutrition Action which you can get at www.cspi.net. I have been a subscriber since 1998).

The consumer is then *educated*, mostly informed and conditioned in how to use them. I make the distinction because I question if we are truly educated when we don't have a fundamental root understanding of how something works. The difference is being able to successfully decode something like nutrition labels to answer the question "how much protein am I really getting from this food source?"

It's not your fault, advertisers and marketers are just very good at their jobs.

So, a consumer advocacy group like CSPI lobbies for nutrition labels and gets them. However, as soon as the nutrition labels were put in place, food manufacturers lobbied congress hard to write legislation that allows for loopholes in nutrition labels by manipulating words and redefining familiar terms.

For example, most of you have been *educated* that the ingredients listed on nutrition labels are listed in order of quantity from most to least. If the 1st ingredient listed is whole wheat flour and the last is sugar, you believe that this food item contains less sugar than any other ingredient listed.

Unfortunately this is not necessarily true.

Congress wrote manufacturers a legislative loophole. Ingredients must be listed in order of quantity **UNLESS** the manufacturer encloses those ingredients in parenthesis, brackets and/or uses a Proprietary Blend of ingredients – Surprise!

This means the consumer has no idea how much of a particular ingredient a food has if it is contained in parenthesis, brackets and/or uses a Proprietary Blend. To be clear, a manufacturer can contain ingredients that are in the least quantity in parenthesis and list them first in the ingredients list giving you the impression these ingredients occur in the greatest quantity when they really do not. This allows the manufacturer to cut in large quantities of cheap, low nutrient ingredients with small fractions of high nutrient ingredients, giving you the impression it is a healthy, nutrient dense food.

This again is why it is crucial you have a rock solid, unshakable model to support your decision making process in order to help you bypass all the games manufacturers and Congress play.

In the chapter named Whole Grains and The Fiber Rule I will explain exactly how to decode and interpret any nutrition label with one simple rule. The Fiber Rule will circumvent any manufacturer and legislative loopholes – period.

Chapter 7

Let's Review

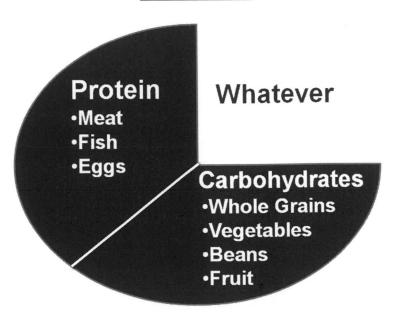

We learned that meat, fish and eggs are the preferred main protein sources because...

- They are complete proteins
- Have high protein start values

To avoid any confusion, "Meat" includes all forms of beef, pork and poultry.

Carbohydrates include:

- Whole Grains – Fiber is 3g or greater per serving.
- Vegetables – Any, but also include dark leafy ones.
- Beans – Legumes and beans of any kind – high fiber.
- Fruit* – Natural sugar/fiber. Most juice has no fiber!

Whatever includes:

- umm...Whatever! – As long as it is in visual proportion to the rest of your protein/carbohydrate choices.

Look, food is a large part of our social dynamic and meant to be enjoyed. So the 1/4 "Whatever" portion is meant to add balance to our eating experience.

Also keep in mind that athletes, especially young athletes need fat in their diet for both general and athletic development. First of all, most competitive athletes can afford the extra calories, fat, etc that low nutrient dense foods like pizza and deserts provide. Second, that 1/4 represents damage control. You can only do so much damage with 25% of your plate while your body is still getting everything it needs from the other 75%.

* Technically, nuts and seeds are fruits. So be aware that many youth programs and facilities ban nuts and many seeds are exposed to nuts during processing.

Chapter 8

Cause and Effect

In the beginning of this book I stated that there are consequences to athletes not eating properly and I will address this now.

Question – Do we get stronger or build up our bodies during sports training, practice or games?

The answer is no, we actually break down our bodies. We lose fluids, carbohydrates, tear muscle fibers and rupture capillaries which cause intracellular bleeding, inflammation and metabolites (waste products). It's not a pretty picture.

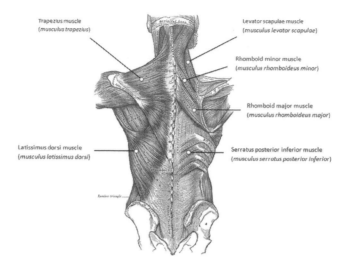

The image above shows muscles of the back, shoulders and neck with skin and fat removed. Below we look deeper inside the muscle to see the actual bundled muscle fibers including nerve and blood supply.

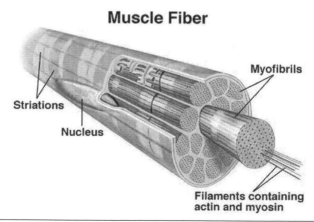

Before Practice   After Practice

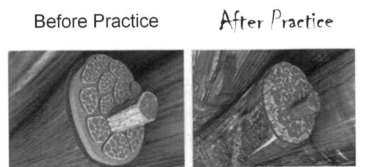

This illustrates what your muscle fibers look like before and after training, especially strength training. The "After" side looks quite degraded as a result of the wear and tear from training.

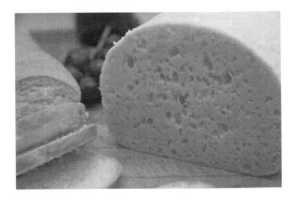

It's similar to Swiss cheese in that we form micro-tears (holes) in our tissues that need to be repaired. It's okay, our bodies were designed to adapt by going through this tearing down and rebuilding process as long as we supply the necessary nutrients to rebuild with.

Why Athletes Need Food

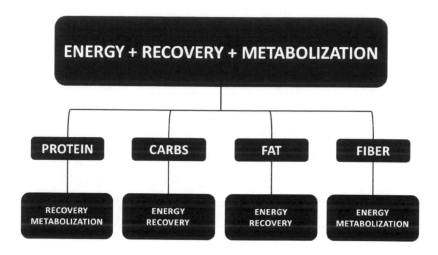

We repair the damage to our tissues with nutrients from our food; in particular, protein, carbohydrates, fat and fiber. These nutrients are metabolized (chemically broken down) and delivered to the damaged tissue via our bloodstream. The body is smart in that it repairs the damaged tissue by making it a bit stronger in case you try assaulting it like that again. This is the basic process of how we become progressively stronger.

The harder you train the more damage you do to your tissue. The greater the damage, the more cellular recovery you need in terms of both time and nutrients. If you do not have proper nutrition to provide the materials for repair, you have a problem.

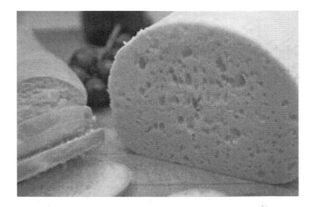

You don't need to know much about the body to realize that micro-tears in your tissue can only serve to weaken the structure and set you up for both acute and chronic injuries as well as poor performance and development.

This is an example of what I commonly hear from both young athletes and their parents. You get home from practice and you "have too much homework" or are "too tired to eat." Perhaps you're one of those families that "doesn't do leftovers" so there is nothing to eat. Then you wake up the next morning for school and don't feel like eating or are running late so you think "I'll just grab a bagel, granola bar or a coffee or just skip it."

Soooooo...how does your body repair the damage!?

This is where it gets interesting...

Chapter 9

Feed Your Body or it will Feed on You!

First of all, by now some of you have heard this concept in different words, but many still have not.

Second, it was October when I initially developed **The 3/4 Rule** as a live presentation for area sports teams. Being moved by the Halloween spirit is how I explain my font choice in the image above.

I'm not kidding, feed your body or it will feed on you. Remember earlier when I said on the cellular level your body does not care about anything other than survival and there are huge consequences if you don't eat Nutrition for Athletes? Well here we go.

Our bodies work on the same cause and effect principle as the rest of our world. So give your body the nutritional material it needs to repair your tissue or it will sacrifice your healthy muscles to get the material it needs.

It's called *catabolism*. This is just a fancy word for destructive metabolism, where your body breaks down your muscle tissue to feed on its protein. Oh you heard right; don't feed your body Nutrition for Athletes and your body will destroy the muscles you spend hours trying to develop each week!

Imagine you are on board a boat that has a hole in the side and it starts taking on water. Rather than getting the proper materials to fix the damage you make a hole in another part of the boat and use that material to effect repairs. Of course you now have to repeat this process to try and repair the damage to the second hole and then the third and so on.

It's pretty easy to see how this process continues to weaken the overall structure of the boat and continues to diminish its abilities and capacity as an athlete, I mean boat – No, I mean athlete.

Why?

Why not Fat or Carbs?

Why does your body sacrifice your muscles instead of stored fat or carbohydrates?

Well that answer is obvious...

Chapter 10

ELECTRICITY!

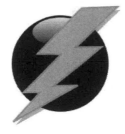

Electricity?

That's right - Electricity!

The current that runs through **The 3/4 Rule** is the foundational principle of electricity. We run on electricity, we are alive because of electricity. Specifically, each heartbeat, every move we make and every thought we create is a result of electro-chemical impulses.

Since our lives literally depend on electricity, do you think perhaps any rule that governs electricity is pretty darn important to us, especially when trying to develop the body?

You better believe it is! As a matter of fact it is the single most important principle in developing the body – period.

So what is this all important principle? What is the primary principle or rule of electricity? Think about this for a moment, most of you know this.

It always takes...

THE PATH OF LEAST RESISTANCE!

That's right; our bodies take the easy way out.

So the answer to the question of why our bodies break down our muscles instead of fat or carbohydrates is because...

It's Easier!

It takes less work and therefore less energy to metabolically break down your muscles tissue for protein than it does to metabolically break down your stored fat or carbohydrate.*

So,

Since your body runs on electricity, all bodily processes operate through "The Path of Least Resistance."

*This specifically refers to the efficiency of accessing stored fat/carbohydrates versus initializing a catabolic process.

CHEW ON THIS!

Now there are always a few minds that want to get caught up in "the thick of thin things" - chew on minutia. Don't spend your time trying to come up with some obscure example or extreme circumstance where this principle might not apply as minor exceptions are irrelevant. An exception does not invalidate a rule; that's what makes it an exception.

Physicists, electrical engineers and electricians – take a breath and relax. The neurophysiologic processes of the body are not the proper context for applications of dielectric breakdowns, Onsager Relations or even the term "electrical current."

Next, don't confuse terms like "path of least resistance" and "easier" with something that is better or smarter. Just because your body reflexively takes the easy path does not mean that path is best for you or your objectives. I point this out as some believe that the body "is smarter than we are" and knows what it needs even if your mind disagrees.

Remember, your nervous system, muscles, tendons, ligaments, organs, etc. all send/receive stimulation and are all governed by one overriding principle – receive and respond to stimulation in the most efficient way possible independent of any plans you may have. Sometimes this is a benefit to you and sometimes it is not.

The Path of Least Resistance

The path used most often puts up the least resistance. This by the way is the process by which we learn everything – good and bad.

The following sequence of images illustrates an easy way to conceptualize this principle with respect to how the body functions.

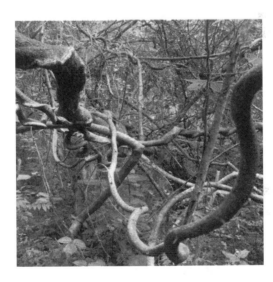

Pictured here is a dense rainforest jungle with no established path where every step requires you to chop vines, plants, move logs and rocks. This requires a lot of time and effort and is an initial dynamic we experience in all areas of life – sports, academics, relationships and occupations.

As we repeat this process, we create a neurological pathway which allows us to communicate our electro-chemical messages more quickly and efficiently, as this pathway offers less resistance with repeated use.

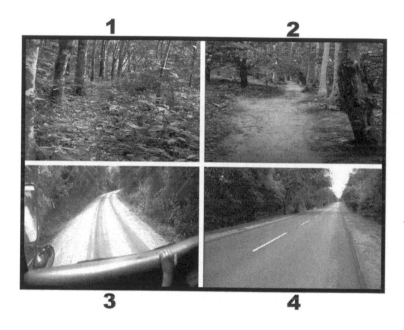

Remember, on the cellular level, your body is indifferent to what things you do. This means if you spend a lot of time practicing correct mathematical formulae, you will get better to some degree in math. And, if you spend a lot of time practicing incorrect mathematical formulae, you will get better to some degree in becoming worse at math.

Huh?

You see, your body is designed to adapt and evolve; essentially to increase its capacity in the specific direction of the stimulation it receives. So you are either getting better at doing something correct, productive, etc., or you are getting better at doing something incorrect, unproductive, etc. We don't get worse at things; we get better at doing things well and better at doing things poorly.

This by the way is how compensations in our bodies occur; we get better at overusing one part of our body which leads to its breakdown – think carpal tunnel.

A drunk becomes better at drinking and better at demonstrating a lack of discipline and self control. Those who practice rude behavior get better at being rude, while those who practice compassion become better at being compassionate. A healthy mind and body do not devolve, they just get better at supporting either positive or negative behavior and development.

If I take a first place youth soccer team and have them practice incorrect skills and incorrect athletic development, they will get better at being a bad team. Since the end result is the same, my soccer team plays worse and wins less, it may feel to you that I am indulging in semantics. However, my point is that the power lies in the distinction of *HOW* you get to the end result from your body's perspective.

The body is designed to adapt and adaptation, in the absence of disease, does not allow you to devolve. This distinction is important because regardless of which pathway we choose, correct/incorrect, productive/unproductive; the outcome is the result in having made that pathway the "Path of Least Resistance."

Similarly, when you practice poor nutrition, your mind and body adapt to make it easier for you to make poor food choices in the future. You get better at eating poorly.

I know, some of you are still scratching your heads and skeptical with this one.

Awesome – Let's continue the discussion online!

Go to www.ChrisWeiler.com/Nutrition

Chapter 11

What have we learned so far!

Nutrition for Survival is not enough for athletic development. Athletes need food for proper energy, recover and metabolization.

¾ of your plate should be filled with protein and carbohydrates from the sources below. The last ¼ of your plate can be filled with whatever you like as long as it is in relative proportion (visual, weight, etc) to the ¾ side.

The ¾ Rule

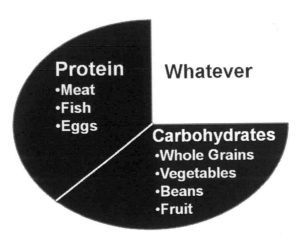

Sports Training Damages Your Body!

So...

> # Feed Your Body
> # or
> # It will Feed on You!

Because of...

ELECTRICITY!

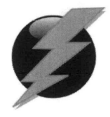

And

The Path of Least
Resistance

Why?

It's Easier to break down your muscles for reconstructive cellular material and energy than stored fat or carbohydrates!

Chapter 12

Vegan. To Be or Not To Be - That is The Question

Earlier I stated reasons why it is challenging to get enough qualified protein as a vegetarian athlete. Now I will briefly offer a few of my thoughts and theories regarding why some vegans can be successful athletes while most cannot.

As is typical with such issues, there are representatives on both sides of the pasture who strongly support their choices. The reality is that there are those who both eat meat and don't eat meat who feel great and compete great.

So how do we reconcile the fact that there are, although not a lot, elite athletes who are strictly vegan? Are they exceptions to the rule? Do they have a unique bio-chemistry and/or metabolism that may or may not be tied to their ethnicity? These are important considerations that require better, more specifically focused research.

However, I believe the most relevant factor is to distinguish between endurance and non-endurance athletes, especially those that strength train. It is not necessary for endurance athletes to train their muscles, tendons and ligaments for maximum strength and power in order to become elite athletes. Conventional wisdom and science both say choose one or the other, as the extent to which you develop one will diminish the other. Train for strength and power, you inhibit endurance development and vice-versa.

Elite vegan athletes who do not eat meat are a minority and the majority of that minority are endurance athletes who don't perform high intensity strength training. This distinction is extremely important in that most sports are not endurance sports, but rather characterized by short bursts of maximum strength, speed and power. However, to be competitive today, non-endurance athletes need to strength train. Soft tissue subject to strength training requires protein to repair and rebuild damaged tissue. If an endurance athlete strength trains at all, it is typically general and not intense enough to warrant much repair/rebuilding.

On the other hand, my daughters friend Azaria is a vegan who is 12 years old, a powerful level 9 gymnast and *shredded* - extremely lean and muscular. Although her training is very demanding, she doesn't eat meat, fish or consume much dairy. Why doesn't she catabolize her muscle tissue? Maybe she does catabolize, but not enough for it to be evident.

Buckle up for this one. Perhaps her unique biochemistry and metabolism is very efficient at sparing nitrogen and/or creates the conditions for a natural anti-catabolic state that mimics the effects of anabolic steroids.

How one *looks* is often misleading as genetic predisposition is often the most powerful influencing factor. The less body fat, the more the underlying shape of your muscles can be seen. Some people have extremely low body fat and can remain lean regardless of what or how they eat. I know, as I am one of those people and I suspect Azaria is as well.

The reality is that genetically gifted athletes thrive despite poor coaching, training, education, environment and nutrition. We have to remember, they are the minority and the exceptions, not the rule.

Furthermore, both endurance (aerobic) and anaerobic athletes are each supported by different energy systems in the body. It is at this level that I would like to see research conducted to discover what I believe is a relationship between a vegan diet and its effect on oxygen uptake, nitrogen, carbon dioxide levels and their metabolization. This research should also test groups that ate vegan and vegan plus meat/fish/dairy protein. This will help answer the question of whether removing animal protein was causal or a substantial increase of vegetables and fruits regardless of what else was eaten.

Personally, I feel my best when I eat meat protein, fruit, vegetables, rice and legumes - typically pinto, black or lentils. However, I don't feel as vital when I leave out the protein or leave out the veggies and legumes - balance.

Share your thoughts and experiences on the vegan issue. Go to www.ChrisWeiler.com/Nutrition or Scan the QR code below with your mobile device.

Chapter 13

Eat More / Eat Less

Eat More	Eat Less
• Protein	• Packaged Food
• Water	• Soda / Fruit Juice
• Whole Grains	• Salt
• Vegetables	• Restaurant / Bakery Food
• Fruits	• Sports drinks

The "Eat More" side of the table is a general restatement of **The 3/4 Rule**. The "Eat Less" side covers the majority of what you should avoid more often than not.

In adopting good policies and rules that govern nutrition for athletes we take the guess work, theory, tips/tricks and marketing out of the equation which greatly simplifies our decision making processes.

It's really just as simple as making sure that most of your food choices fit into the "Eat More" side and you're covered. The power in the nutrition policy of **The 3/4 Rule** is that it is specific enough to guide you through each meal, yet broad enough to rely on in the future and at any location you may find yourself needing to eat.

What to eat before and/or during training

YES	NO
• Granola – bars, mix, etc.	• Soda / Fruit Juice
• Protein	• Sports drinks
• Whole Grains	• Candy / Cookies / Donuts
• Vegetables	
• Fruits	
• Water	

In our overscheduled society, the reality is that many kids need to eat on the run between school, activities and sports practice.

Therefore, this table more specifically targets how to eat and how not to eat before and/or during training.

Every athlete needs to listen to their gut and learn from experience how much to eat before and/or during training. The volume or quantity of food eaten is not important. Following **The 3/4 Rule** is important.

Eating (snacking) during training is dependent on each athlete's tolerance and sport. Most athletes don't have a problem taking a bite or two of granola or banana during their hydration breaks. Swimming tends to be an issue as many pools/coaches have rules about food near the pool.

The Rules about eating during training

- After around 90 minutes of continuous, intense training most everyone has depleted their stored energy from food, so it makes sense to replenish sometime before you run out of fuel.

- However, the problem is that I rarely see young athletes exceeding this 90 minute mark. Just because a team may have practice for 2-4 hours, doesn't mean that every individual is working intensely for over 90 minutes. Typically each athlete's net training is something less.

- The body's ability to store energy is finite and how much you eat or what you eat does not change that capacity. Therefore trying to *pre-load* your body with a sports drink before practice/training is rarely useful.

- If you do not feed your body with some type of carbohydrate (protein would be helpful too)
  - Your training will suffer.
  - Increase chances for acute/chronic injuries.
  - You will enter into *catabolism* (destructive metabolism)
  - Slow your recovery/recuperation.

- Avoid this typical scenario. You don't follow The 3/4 Rule, so you have energy (sugar) highs and lows throughout the day. The sports drink or energy drink gives you that quick energy surge so it becomes a habit. Due to poor eating habits, your energy is low at the end of school, so you need another sugar rush before practice.

- For most athletes drinking a lot of sports drinks will not help; drinking small amounts will help. 6 to 12 ounces diluted with 50% water is sufficient for the majority of athletes in most climates. The sports drink, like any tool, requires thoughtful, proper application. However, every day I see athletes drinking them on the way to school, before, during and after practice as well as when hanging out with friends. The sports drink is a highly concentrated form of sugar and electrolytes - period. For most athletes a little during and after practice is more than enough.

- While it's true that consuming a sports drink before practice can help deliver energy to working muscles so as to help spare muscles from entering a catabolic cycle, that's not the whole story. We need to make sure we are not sacrificing proper nutrition during the day and entering an addictive cycle using an energy drink as a quick patch to get us through practice. That is a recipe for poor development and bad habits.

It is important to understand supplements in their proper context. Typically, a supplement might fill in a few cracks in your nutritional foundation. You have been training for 2 hours, used up all your energy stores and are becoming catabolic. Taking a few bites of fruit, granola, yogurt, or ingesting a sports drink or gel will fill in some of those metabolic *cracks* and help address catabolism.

Let me be clear, when you have exhausted your stored energy supplies and your body starts to slow down, hit the wall, bonk, crash, etc., this is in part because you have run out of fuel and in part because catabolism is an inefficient metabolic process in terms of giving you energy for training. It's a weak substitute.

So yes, you can push your body to the point of breaking and win a competition or game in a catabolic state – that's okay. But you cannot consistently train this way without future consequences.

Chapter 14

Whole Grains & The Fiber Rule

The simplicity and power of The Fiber Rule

While water, protein, fruits and vegetables are easy to recognize, many people find it challenging to identify whole grains. This challenge is usually compounded by confusing marketing and advertising claims such as "whole grains", multi-grain, "whole wheat", "stone ground", "8 grains", "wheat flour", etc.

Do you know the difference between "wheat flour" and "whole wheat flour?" Let's be honest, many of you don't care to be educated in the differences, you care about the result. When you look at the nutrition label, you want to easily identify if it is a nutrient dense food or not.

In this section we will cut through all the marketing misdirection and I will teach you exactly how to evaluate any food item with a nutrition label.

I call it "Whole Grains and The Fiber Rule."

The Fiber Rule is your secret weapon that enables you to know without a doubt whether or not the ingredients are really whole grains.

There is a relationship between the ingredients list and the amount of fiber listed under the Nutrition Facts table. If the dietary fiber serving is 3 grams or above, 2 grams for crackers or any crunchy carbohydrate that comes in a bag, you can be confident that you have a quality, whole grain food source.

The more grams of fiber per serving means that a higher percentage of the food you are eating comes from whole grains. If you are eating a piece of bread that has 2 grams of fiber per serving versus one that has 6 grams per serving, you know that the 2 gram slice of bread contains a low amount of whole grain ingredients and is therefore, not as nutrient dense.

The ideal range of fiber you are looking for is 3-12 grams per serving. Whole wheat is the most common defining characteristic of a high fiber grain. This is why a package of pasta made from enriched flour has 1 or 2 grams of fiber and pasta made from whole wheat flour has 5 or 6 grams per serving.

CHEW ON THIS!

The higher the fiber content the more nutritious your food is.

Since the fiber content is the defining measure of a whole grain, don't even bother reading the marketing claims on the package; simply look at the fiber content.

It's just that simple. To test for whole grains in the picture below, simply look at the fiber content – 10 grams! That's huge and well above our minimum 3 grams per serving.

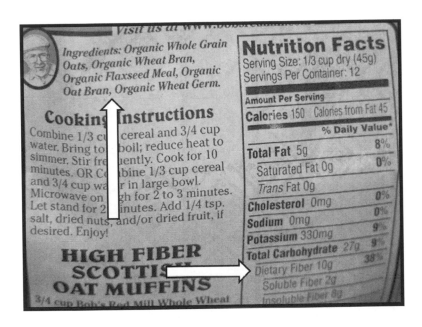

In the magnified picture below, I have combined both the ingredients and fiber listing for easier viewing. We can be absolutely confident that this food is made from whole grains.

Note 1: Although there is often a relationship, *organic* ingredients are not required for high fiber and whole grains.

Note 2: You only need to focus on the "Dietary Fiber" amount. Don't worry about "Soluble" (breaks down in water) or "Insoluble" fiber (does not break down in water). In following The ¾ Rule you will get all your fiber needs met automatically. Again, this is the value of using a powerful nutrition model.

INGREDIENTS: Organic Whole Grain Oats, Organic Wheat Bran, Organic Flaxseed Meal, Organic Oat Bran, Organic Wheat Germ.

Manufactured in a facility that uses tree nuts, soy, wheat and milk.

Potassium 330mg	**9%**
Total Carbohydrate 27g	**9%**
Dietary Fiber 10g ⬅	**38%**
Soluble Fiber 2g	

Let's test your understanding of The Fiber Rule!

Look at the image below. What Do You Think?

RAMEN NOODLE INGREDIENTS:
ENRICHED WHEAT FLOUR (WHEAT FLOUR, NIACIN, REDUCED IRON, THIAMINE MONONITRATE, RIBOFLAVIN, FOLIC ACID), VEGETABLE OIL (CONTAINS ONE OR MORE OF THE FOLLOWING: CANOLA, COTTONSEED, PALM) PRESERVED BY TBHG, CONTAINS LESS THAN 1% OF :SALT, SOY SAUCE (WATER, WHEAT, SOYBEANS, SALT), POTASSIUM CARBONATE, SODIUM (MONO, HEXAMETA, AND/OR TRIPOLY) PHOSPHATE, SODIUM CARBONATE, TURMERIC.

To test for whole grains apply The Fiber Rule by first looking at the ingredients list. Here we find "enriched wheat flour" listed first and need to determine if this is a whole grain.

As a rule if you see the word "enriched" don't waste your time; put it back on the shelf and move on. Enriched means the nutrients, including fiber have been processed out and then artificially added back in, typically with lower quality vitamins than occur naturally in the food. As the FDA does not require the fiber to be added back in during the enrichment process, it is not and therefore lost.

However, if you are unsure look at the fiber content, which gives you a complete picture of this foods nutritional value.

One gram of fiber is not a worthwhile grain.

It gets even worse when we look at the rest of the nutritional breakdown.

By percentage, from most to least this food primarily delivers:

1. Sodium – 35%
2. Saturated Fat – 18%
3. Total Fat – 11%
4. Total Carbohydrates – 9% (not whole grain)

Amount Per Serving	%DV*	Amount Per Serving	%DV*
Total Fat 7g	**11%**	**Total Carbohydrate** 26g	**9%**
Saturated Fat 3.5g	**18%**	Dietary Fiber 1g	**4%**
Trans Fat 0g		Sugars 1g	
Cholesterol 0mg	**0%**	**Protein** 5g	
Sodium 830mg	**35%**		
Vitamin A** • Vitamin C	0%	• Calcium** • Iron	

If you want to see more examples of The Fiber Rule in action go to my website: www.ChrisWeiler.com/Nutrition

Chapter 15

WHAT ABOUT SUPPLEMENTS?

Those unregulated, expensive, heavily marketed magic bullets that promise to make us bigger, stronger, faster, feel more energized, lose weight, gain weight or in some way give us that competitive edge.

Although with an introduction like that, it sounds like I am quite biased and against the use of supplements – I'm not. I do however need to put supplements in the correct context for your proper digestion – both figurative and literal.

First of all, the way we have been conditioned through marketing/advertising to relate to supplements violates the root principle of my Performance Model – The *thing* Has No Power! That sports drink, powder, pill (legal) has no power to give you anything by itself. It's just a tool in your toolbox that if used at the wrong time or in the wrong way will not help you achieve your sports performance objectives.

Second, if you use them, then by definition they should *supplement* your real food eating plan. A supplement should fill in the gaps that exist in your real food diet.

EXAMPLES

For whatever reason, you have not eaten since lunch and cannot eat before practice/training/game hours later – the supplement tool may be a smart choice. Perhaps you can't stomach food in the morning, which means it's a supplement or nothing until lunch – the supplement tool may be a smart choice.

The reality is that most supplements run the range from useless/harmless to useful, with most of them clustered at the useless/harmless end of the spectrum.

HOW TO USE SUPPLEMENTS – The smart way

This discussion will be limited to supplements that can be purchased legally.

First, let's categorize supplements:

1. Recovery
2. Energy/Ergogenic Aid

Recovery

- You just practiced/trained for 1 or more hours and for whatever reason are unable to eat. Remembering the Nutrition for Athletes Model you know you need to give your body the nutritional building blocks to aid in recovery of your tissues or your body will begin to catabolize your muscle tissue for this energy. Therefore a protein or protein/carbohydrate supplement would be the smart choice. Now, in the absence of any quality protein supplement, this would be the time to dig through your nutrition tool box and if available drink some milk (yes even chocolate) and drink it applying the *it's better than nothing* principle.

Energy/Ergogenic Aids

- Sports/energy drinks and creatine are commonly used examples. In context of our discussion here, "Ergogenic" is just fancy word for a supplement that enhances performance.

Common reasons for use

- Too little sleep, too much sleep, sick, injured, sore, poor eating habits (not following The ¾ Rule) and/or you're a teenager and through no fault of your own are a raging mess of hormones that cause wild fluctuations in your energy levels.

- Ignorance – If the internet or the bottle says it works, it must be true.

- Fear – Not confident that you alone, without aid, are good enough.

- Ultra Competitive – Looking for any edge.

- Cheat/Shortcut Mentality – Looking for any edge.

- Placebo Effect – You need a security blanket. It doesn't matter whether the supplement actually works or not as long as you believe it can positively affect your performance.

- Addiction/Dependence – Through consistent use/abuse you have conditioned your body and mind to need the highly caffeinated and/or sugary beverage in order to just feel *normal*.

VITAMINS

"These statements have not been evaluated by the Food and Drug Administration. This product is not intended to diagnose, treat, cure or prevent any disease."

Every vitamin and mineral sold is a supplement, which means it must have the above quoted language printed on its label.

What you need to understand about Vitamins and Minerals:

1. There are good arguments to support both taking and not taking a daily multi-vitamin supplement. My thinking is you could take one 1 – 4 days per week.

Why?

- The average person consumes a high percentage of processed and fast foods; both of which lack nutrient density.

- Many fresh produce items are sourced from outside the United States or outside the region you live in. As a result, they lose much of their nutrients during the process of shipping, sitting in the grocery store and finally waiting in your home until consumed.

2. When a supplement like vitamins appear to have some potential benefit, yet lack regulation or conclusive proof, I like to apply the first law of toxicology - "The dose makes the poison." This means all things are toxic in high enough doses - including water. The idea is to keep intake levels high enough to provide some benefit, but low enough to avoid harm. By not taking a multi-vitamin every day, you allow your body to more fully metabolize the vitamin, which helps minimize it's build up in your body.

3. As a supplement, vitamins are not regulated by the FDA.

This means

- No assurances of quality, quantity, potency, or accuracy of any ingredients in your vitamin or mineral tablet, gel, powder or drink.

- Look closely at DV% - Daily Value. Many vitamins have hundreds to thousands percent greater potency per serving above the recommended DV. For example, right now I am looking at the label of a daily vitamin supplement and it lists Thiamin at 1667% of DV. Even if you are able to metabolize 50% of this amount it is still likely much more than you need to ingest daily.

Another issue is that most vitamin supplements are manufactured in a lab which means they are not a whole food with a fully intact nutrient profile – they are a synthetic. Vitamin supplements use *isolated fractions* of vitamins that occur naturally in the whole food and therefore need the co-factors normally found in the whole food in order to fully complete its chemical processing.

Think of this process as ingredients in a cookie recipe. If you leave out a key ingredient or two, you will bake something other than a fully intact cookie.

This means vitamin supplements do not work alone and need food to be properly metabolized. Stop for a minute and think about how this impacts the value of vitamins and supplements in the form of pills, water, gum, gels, etc. The takeaway is that vitamin supplements are not that helpful unless digested with food.

Dr. David Katz, director of the Yale University Prevention Research Center, said the main problems with taking supplements are uncertainties and misunderstandings about the proper dose and combination of these vitamins.

"We know that nutrients are beneficial in foods, but divorced of that context, and packaged somewhat 'arbitrarily' by us, the effects may be very different," Katz said. "Imagine if you had all the right materials to build a house but in all the wrong proportions, and then tried to put together a well-built house."

For most people, taking a multi-vitamin supplement 1-4 times per week will not cause any harm. This balanced approach provides an opportunity to benefit from vitamins/minerals that you may be deficient in, while keeping your total weekly intake levels below the over-fortification threshold.

Think of taking a vitamin as applying a liquid sealant on the foundation of your home. You don't know how many micro cracks, crevices, gaps or holes the foundation has, but know that a sealant will fill in more of them than if you had not applied it.

Remember, every individual has their own unique genetic, biological, physiological, neurological and metabolic markers, variances, tolerances, considerations and predispositions. Therefore, you should FIRST always consult with your medical doctor to make sure any supplement is not contraindicated for you specifically.

If you track research in this or most any industry, you will find that in the next 6 months to 5 years, much of what research has "proven" today will be "disproven" and replaced by the next research flavor of the moment that has been "proven" until that is replaced and the cycle repeats. I point this out as the fitness/sports training industry is in a current love affair with "evidence based research/training" and mistakenly holds it up as the final word on a given subject - It's not. At best it's only the beginning and that's if it's conducted properly - mostly it's not.

Research is often flawed in 3 ways: First, the inability to go wide and deep. There is an inverse relationship between the number of variables involved in an experiment and its probability for valid results. As the variables increase, so do the chances for error.

Second, by asking the wrong question(s). If you ask the wrong question, you will get the wrong answer. How you conduct your research, i.e. correct protocol, use and application of correct formulae can all be valid, but ask the wrong question(s), your results will be invalid and your conclusions false.

Third, poor test tools and/or subjects. Some physicians still cite height/weight and BMI norms. However, many fail to tell you that these formulae and tables are based on the "Average American in apparently healthy condition." I have never met this person and neither have you. More to the point, these numbers, normative values and averages are NOT based on athletic youth.

This again is why it is important to apply models of *How* you do things, as they are what stands strong against the ever changing winds of research.

The Piper Must be Paid

There are some that claim that you can trick the body by artificially inducing the digestive process through mastication (chewing). As a matter of fact, there used to be a short lived trend of chewing a piece of meat to extract its flavor and provide the catalyst for the digestive process, but spitting it out without swallowing to avoid the caloric impact of the food. It was difficult for this trend to gain traction as it was hard for image conscience people to reconcile the fantasy of eating with zero caloric impact while spitting their food into a napkin during meals – pretty gross.

While it is true that the act of chewing ignites a chemical chain reaction that gets the digestive juices flowing, salivation, digestive enzymes/acids, etc, the body cannot be fooled for long. Your stomach and associated digestive chemicals have prepared the digestive environment for metabolization which requires something to metabolize – food.

At this point your body has options. The digestive juices could simply get reabsorbed back into your system and maybe you feel a little acid rumbling in your stomach. However, your body also has the option of metabolizing whatever is most readily available as the digestive environment has already been prepared and just needs to pull something in to digest.

If we apply what we learned about the path of least resistance, we realize that one's body could choose to sacrifice some muscle tissue to complete the already activated digestive process. Each individual's unique metabolic biochemistry will determine which option is exercised.

Now that we are armed with a better understanding on how to think about digestion and metabolization, it's pretty easy to understand just how useless "Vitamin Gum" is.

- Vitamins cannot be fully metabolized without food.
- Begins digestive process, but provides nothing to digest.
- May create the causes for the body to catabolize muscle tissue.

While speaking on vitamin supplement use to WebMD, David Katz, MD, MPH, director of the Yale University Prevention Research Center whose medical practice specializes in nutrition states, "What I'm more likely to see is a person with a dosing level of supplements that's higher than optimal."

Scientists don't yet know if routinely getting a little bit too much of a vitamin or mineral (as opposed to a mega dose) is a problem, Katz says.

"There might be hints of concern, but they would be very subtle signs," he says.

"These fairly mild symptoms may include difficulty sleeping or concentrating, nerve problems such as numbness or tingling, or feeling more irritable – depending on the nutrient that's going overboard."

Katz states that a bigger concern is that we're "garnishing the food supply with over-fortification."

"When more and more foods are enhanced, it becomes impossible for consumers to know what dose they're getting over the course of a day," says Katz. "Clinicians have to realize we might be introducing new dietary imbalances because of this practice."

The power for the consumer is in "How" we think about supplements. Most supplements are harmless to the majority of (not all) people. More often than not, the supplement only serves to lighten your wallet.

Protein, carbohydrate, creatine, chondroitin and glucosamine all fall into this category. It gets more complicated when we are talking about 5htc and any of the other supplements that can directly affect your brains neurotransmitter and hormone levels.

Says biochemist Dr. Michael Colgan, "Neurotransmitters are the chemicals that carry information from one nerve to another. Their activity constitutes your mind, your consciousness, all your schemes and dreams. So before you mess with them you better know what you are doing."

Keep this in mind regarding supplements.

- Do you know if you have enough or not?
  - Unless you have specialized blood work performed, you have no idea whether you have too much or too little of any given vitamin, mineral, enzyme and/or hormone.
- Am I a member of the "At Risk" population?
  - Diseases/Disorders or family history of the immune, respiratory, digestive, metabolic, neurological, circulatory systems, etc.
  - Very young or old populations.

Here's what you can count on:

- The medical community makes discoveries either through specific research or serendipitous occurrence.

- The popular press will feed those discoveries to the public often citing results and promoting claims without proper context.

- Supplement manufacturers will begin marketing products based on that research, again usually out of context.

- Sometime in the next 6 to 24 months, new discoveries and research will *disprove* them and supplant them with something new.

- Manufacturers now redirect the public to yet another part of the pasture to graze on the new supplement.

Real world examples:

- Vitamin E is good...the market moves on Vitamin E.
- Vitamin E is bad...the market moves off Vitamin E.
  - Vitamin A
  - Vitamin D
  - Vitamin B-Complex
  - Fish oil - Omega 3's
  - Acai
  - Ginko
  - Selenium
  - Raspberry Ketone
- The list goes on and the herd goes "Moo."

However, it doesn't stop there. Check out this tricky sleight of hand. Supplement manufacturers also like to get mid research findings. This means that at any point during the research continuum you would look for any positive results to support a conclusion in the supplement you want to promote.

Let's say a 5 year research study is underway on CoQ10 (Coenzyme Q10). Preliminary findings at the 1 year mark show CoQ10 effective at sparing lean muscle tissue. Although the study is still 4 years away from its conclusion and still a long way off from understanding negative side effects, the manufacturer begins manufacturing and selling CoQ10 by stating that it "Builds lean muscle tissue and metabolizes fat."

This being a very loose and premature extrapolation of the preliminary findings "CoQ10 spares lean muscle tissue."

Four years later the study concludes and its results do not support the preliminary findings. What happens now is interesting as this is where capitalism and ethics cross paths. You see the manufacturer has a warehouse full of CoQ10 that the study concluded does not support its claims and now has a choice to make regarding their CoQ10 asset.

Choice 1 – stop sales of CoQ10 and lose invested money and future profits associated with that product.

Choice 2 – simply find other research that supports your product, even if you have to *customize* its findings so it supports your products claims.

In the case of CoQ10, this particular manufacturer cited an obscure medical finding that "CoQ10 spares lean muscle tissue and increases fat metabolization" to support its product pitch that it will help you lose fat and gain muscle. This enabled it to continue to sell its stockpile of product.

The manufacturer pulled a crafty editing job on the medical reference regarding CoQ10.

Below is a summary of what the public did not see.

A burn unit ward in a Russian hospital found that burn victims with 70% or more burn coverage who were on life support, being fed intravenously, in a state of accelerated atrophy and muscle wasting, "Spared more lean muscle tissue when given CoQ10."

That is a very specific set of isolated criteria for CoQ10 to be effective under and has little, if anything to do with the effects on healthy bodies not on life support and not suffering from extreme atrophy and muscle wasting.

It's not uncommon for supplement manufacturers to support their product claims with obscure research that is barely linked to its original source or conditions. Most often mouse studies are cited as the only evidence to support supplement claims. I think that the average person (majority) does not know that mouse studies (rodent testing) have a very low correlation to human efficacy. This means *valid* mouse studies mostly turn out results that are *not valid* on humans. Mouse studies are where research starts, not ends. If all you have are results from mouse studies then you cannot conclude anything regarding results on humans.

This is exactly why the FDA has such a rigorous and lengthy process involved with screening medications. It takes time and proper scientific scrutiny to determine the relevant and irrelevant factors that support manufacturers claims.

My *Model* (rules and guidelines) for nutrition and supplements goes like this.

1. FACT: Supplements are not regulated which means the manufacturer does not have to prove it does anything.

2. FACT: Supplement manufacturers have a long history of finding obscure tests/research that cannot be duplicated, is not performed on humans or they edit the research text and then weave the edited bits into a marketing piece in support of their claims.

3. FACT: Within the next 6 months to 2 years, the majority of what the medical community claims as fact about nutrition or supplements will be *proven* wrong and replaced by the next flavor of the moment supported by the same shoddy research. When this happens, manufacturers will push their new product and key influential people in the media and online will direct the herd to graze in another part of pasture where they can now buy new products that are not any more effective than the ones they replaced. In the next 6 months to 2 years this process will repeat itself over again as the herd, the public, will be kept moving back and forth from one side of the pasture to the other – Moo!

Remember, supplement manufacturers can produce and claim what they like; even filling their bottles with useless ingredients. My favorite supplement infomercial of all time was called "Exercise in a Bottle." *"Don't waste your time exercising, when you can get the same exercise benefits while you sleep with Exercise in a Bottle."* That's right, a magic pill you take to get fit while you sleep! Brilliantly crafted language designed to excite our cultural magic bullet mentality.

I'll say it again, The *thing* Has No Power - You Do!

So let's keep it simple by following these rules.

A whey protein isolate or concentrate powdered protein is a smart choice before, during and/or after training.

- Yes, creatine is a scientifically supported ergogenic aid. I am not suggesting you use or don't use it, as it can have low level gastric side effects in some individuals. Just know that it is backed by peer-reviewed research that supports its claims. Questions? Go to at www.ChrisWeiler.com/Nutrition

- Most young athletes should greatly reduce their sports drink intake as most have not trained hard or long enough to require their use. That means 90 minutes or more of continuous, hard training. Not the time your entire team trains as a whole, but you personally. However, for those athletes that do require a sports drink, most don't need more than 4-8 ounces diluted up to 50% as most are highly concentrated.

- A multi-vitamin supplement taken 1-4 times per week is suggested, especially if you don't regularly eat a whole food diet.

Chapter 16

CHEW ON THIS!

Tasty nuggets of wisdom from The 3/4 Rule all in one place.

- Can you apply **The 3/4 Rule** to every meal, of course not. However, you can always keep it in mind and apply it as often as possible.

- Remember, **The 3/4 Rule** is a flexible framework in "How" to eat for optimum athletic development. This means it can easily be used and applied by everyone without requiring unrealistic eating habits that cannot be maintained.

- The ¾ Rule is a tool and as such the skill in which you apply this tool is dependent on your intentions. Your mind guides how you use the tool, which in turn determines the quality of what you are trying to build. If you have a self-defeating perspective then you will be looking for opportunities and excuses to not use the tool correctly and therefore not achieve your objectives.

- It's not a requirement that you fill the last 1/4 of your plate with some nutritionally bankrupt, artificially flavored, sugar packed food. You could fill it with something nutritious or nothing at all.

- To be clear, drink all the milk you want, bathe in it if you like, I just don't recommend it as one of your main protein sources to support Nutrition for Athletes.
  - Low protein start-value.
  - Most people do not consume enough to compensate for the low protein start value.

- There are always a few minds that want to get caught up in "the thick of thin things" (chew on minutia) – Don't. Simply follow The 3/4 Rule.

- Remember, your nervous system, muscles, tendons, ligaments, organs, etc. all send/receive stimulation and are all governed by one overriding principle – receive and respond to stimulation in the most efficient way possible independent of any plans you may have.

- The higher the fiber content the more nutritious your food is.

Now I want to hear from

YOU!

Although the focus of this book is about how young athletes should eat, **The 3/4 Rule** applies to most people of any age - including you. I'm sure many of you have questions about food allergies, weight loss, energy, etc. Did you know pork is metabolized as a red meat or milk actually increases stomach acid not buffer it? And there is much to discuss about buying organic, pasture-fed, vegetable-fed or grain-fed meat and dairy.

You will always have more questions that go beyond the scope of any book. So the format for presentation, the book, is static while the subject and YOU are dynamic.

Let's Get DYNAMIC!

Meet me at www.ChrisWeiler.com/Nutrition

We'll take this discussion to a whole new level. Ask your questions and share your experiences as we help each other improve the quality of our lives and the development of our youth. I'll also be posting dates and times for live discussions and Q&A. And since my Performance Model is about the complete development of young athletes, ALL areas of physical and mental development will be addressed.

I really look forward to seeing you there!

About the Author

Although you may not know me yet, I am about to turn the world of youth sports training right side up.

On the surface a background in philosophy and physics may seem... well... "Interesting", it inadvertently helped provide a foundation for the development of my unique perspectives in athletic development and rehabilitation.

I don't just ask the questions and point out problems most others don't – I also bring solutions.

I enjoy my family, kayaking, rock climbing, 4 wheeling off-road, Buddhism, burning the midnight oil, problem solving and pie. My literary heroic thinkers are Isaac Asimov, Steven Covey, Aldous Huxley, William James, Steven Levitt, George Orwell, Ayn Rand, Socrates and Dr. Seuss.

Did I mention pie?

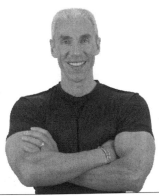

Made in the USA
San Bernardino, CA
22 December 2014